D1827422

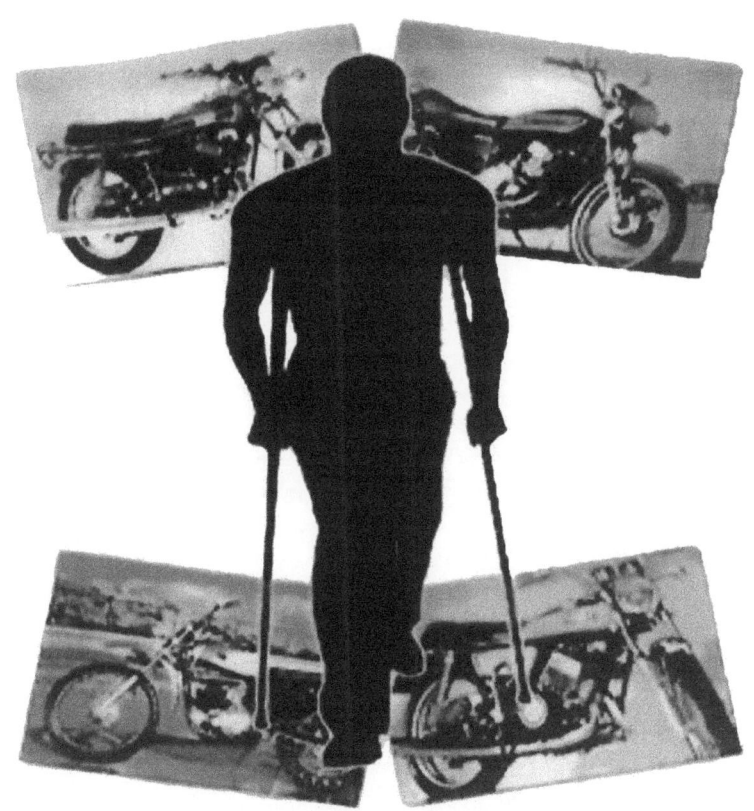

N I G E L   J O H N   B O L T O N

ONE
STEP
AT A TIME

authorHOUSE®

AuthorHouse™ UK
1663 Liberty Drive
Bloomington, IN 47403 USA
www.authorhouse.co.uk
Phone: UK TFN: 0800 0148641 (Toll Free inside the UK)
*   UK Local: (02) 0369 56322 (+44 20 3695 6322 from outside the UK)*

© 2022 Nigel John Bolton. All rights reserved.

No part of this book may be reproduced, stored in a retrieval system, or transmitted by any means without the written permission of the author.

Published by AuthorHouse 12/16/2021

ISBN: 978-1-6655-9560-5 (sc)
ISBN: 978-1-6655-9559-9 (e)

Print information available on the last page.

Any people depicted in stock imagery provided by Getty Images are models, and such images are being used for illustrative purposes only. Certain stock imagery © Getty Images.

This book is printed on acid-free paper.

Because of the dynamic nature of the Internet, any web addresses or links contained in this book may have changed since publication and may no longer be valid. The views expressed in this work are solely those of the author and do not necessarily reflect the views of the publisher, and the publisher hereby disclaims any responsibility for them.

CONTENTS

INTRODUCTION

This is the true story of how my passion for motorbikes nearly killed me and subsequently changed my entire life.

After the last accident I suffered from a Hemiparesis (A traumatic brain injury). I was left with life changing problems especially with my mobility. The biggest problem I had was, should I listen to what the specialists had to say, or should I ignore them and fight it anyway? (No contest) I was going to fight it.

Up to now it's a fight that has lasted 42 years, and I'm still fighting it. I will be the first to admit that it hasn't been easy, far from it, but what I have achieved has far surpassed anything I could have hoped for. Not only did I fight the specialists, I fought the system, a system which seems to be geared up to make life a lot harder for those who want to try. It seems to me that you get a lot more out of the system if you sit back on your bum and do sod all.

I wanted more than that, I wanted my life and my mobility back. There have been lots of ups and downs along the way, as well as four marriages, but giving in was never an option, not then, not now and not ever.

IN THE BEGINNING

The year was 1972 and I had just left school. I started work at Storthes Hall Hospital, Kirkburton nr Huddersfield, which was a very old Victorian mental hospital, set in its own grounds. It was totally self-sufficient with its own farm, plasterers, plumbers, painters, electricians and fire brigade, as well as its own bakery, butchers' shop and shopping department which also had a tailor's shop in it. In the hospital there were a couple of shops and a pub for the patients called The Toby Jug.

I soon settled into work and all that it entailed, as I knew most of the staff already as my dad had worked there for years, and now he was my boss. I started as a trainee assistant chef and really enjoyed it. As part of the training, I had to spend time in each department in and around the kitchen. One of the best places to work was the butchers shop, where I learnt how bone out and prepare meat for the next day, and you got to work with Paul Mellor, who was also a keen biker and did motocross most weekends, he always had a story to tell about biking and the isle of man TT.

I was always keen to listen, and it wasn't long before I was spending most evenings in his workshop learning how he prepared his Greaves moto crosser ready for his next race. His brother Phil was also a biker who at the time had a Yamaha YR5 and a lot of nights he would take me home on it (not for the faint hearted) he could really ride a motorbike.

As time went by it wasn't long before I bought a 250cc Greaves Challenger, which I kept at my dad's farm out in the sticks, as he had a lot of land I could ride on and also a barn where I could store the bike.

The bike was brilliant but it wasn't long before I was looking for something better and that's when I ended up with a Greaves 380 QUB, but deep down all I wanted was a road bike of my own and my own independence. The big day finally arrived, it was the 26th of November, my birthday and I was now 17 and could get a driving licence and a road bike. I soon started looking but the ones I could afford I didn't like and the ones I liked I couldn't afford, Bummer or what? One day on our way home from work dad asked how the search for a bike was going, "not so good" I replied, "Oh well" said dad "something will turn up", then headed towards town, "where are you going" I asked, "well I thought we could go and look around some of the bike dealers in town and see what they have", "oh yes" I replied excitedly "that's a brilliant idea, let's start at Moores the Honda dealer", and that's exactly what we did.

After a good hunt around there was nothing in my price range so we headed down to Earnshaw's on Manchester Road who had some lovely bikes in, there was a Suzuki GT 250 in first class condition but sadly was way too expensive for my pocket, so we made our way around to Smithies at Lockwood. As we pulled up outside the shop, there was the man himself, John Smith, "now then lads, what can I do for you?" he asked, I started to explain what I was looking for and how much I had to spend, when he said "I've got just the bike for you my lad" and led me around to the workshop.

In the workshop was Bud the mechanic working on some old scooter, "and what you after" he asked, Smithie said "show them that yam that came in last week", "ok" said Bud as he started moving bikes around, then wheeled out a Yamaha 250 YDS7, oh yes that's just what I've been looking for, "can I take it for a blast?", "sure you can" he replied and then started it up.

I was soon flying around the block, after about 10 minutes I drove it back to the workshop where Smithie asked me what I thought, "I will have it" I replied, "depending on the price", "ok" he said and started scribbling numbers down on a bit of paper. "It's yours for £200 and I will service it as well", "it's a deal" I replied and handed over the money. "When can I pick it up" I asked, "I will service it in the morning and you can pick it up around 4pm, if that's ok with you?", "that's just fine" I replied. I climbed back into the car and headed for home, now the proud owner of a GDP70L.

As we got closer to home dad commented on what a good bike it was for the money and that I just had to get it insured in the morning, "yep I know, I will do it first thing" I replied, "ok" said dad "but there is one thing you have forgotten about", "what's that?" I asked, "you still have to tell your mother" (ummm, I was just thinking about that, as mum wasn't a big fan of motorbikes at all). The first thing I did when I got in was tell her what I had just bought but before I could finish, she had guessed and went off on one at both of us. It's the lad's choice but she still wasn't having any of it and wouldn't listen to what we had to say. I got the silent treatment for a couple of days, but I could live with that. It was a small price to pay for what was going to be sat in the garage tomorrow.

The next day at work really dragged but as soon as the clock hit 3pm I was off, dad gave me a lift to Lockwood to pick it up, as well as the third degree about speeding and being responsible and not giving my mother anything else to moan about.

We were soon at Smithies and as we pulled up outside, there was the bike, all washed, polished and shiny. "Here you are lad" said Smithie "It's all yours". I couldn't get my helmet on quick enough when he gave me the keys and I was soon heading towards Castle Hill then down Storthes Hall Lane then home.

I pulled up outside the house and mum and came out, "sounds nice" said dad, "yep, sure does" I replied as I popped it on its side stand, but mum just shook her head and walked back into the house.

The next morning, I was up and about very early and soon had the bike out of the garage and was setting off for work. The day went on forever but at last it was home time and there was no holding me back. When I got home my tea was ready which I bolted down and I was off, I went straight to Shelley to show to the bike to Paul and Phil who both thought I had a good deal, but Paul still wheeled it into his workshop and gave it the once over.

The months were flying by and it wasn't long before it was bike test day, which in them days was totally different to how they do it now. I passed my test and over the next twelve months I went all over, Caldwell, Mallory and Brands.

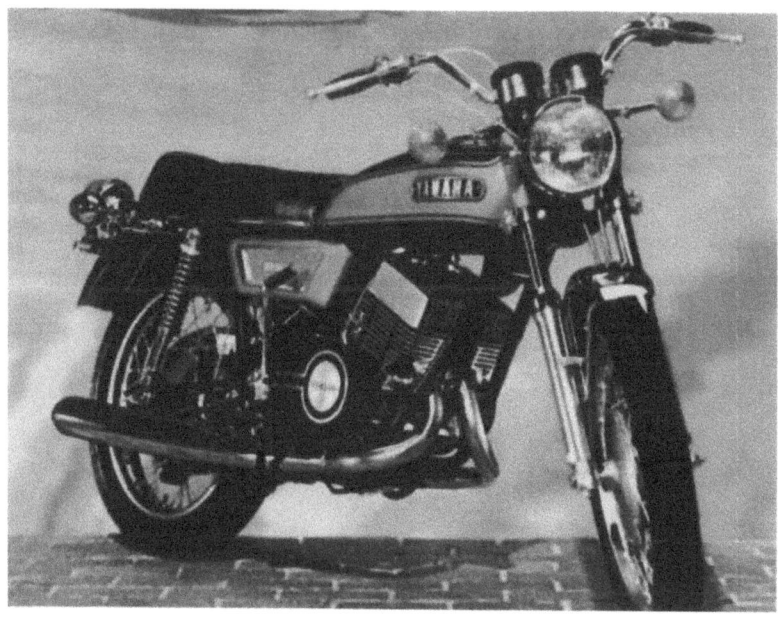

I loved the bike, but Yamaha had just brought out the new RD range and as soon as I had seen the new RD 350, I wanted one. I was soon on my way to Silvester's in Holmfirth to order one. Two weeks later I was on my way back to Silvester's to pick up my new RD 350, it was metallic purple and a good looking bike and had all the latest kit on it, reed valve and disc brakes were fitted as standard, which back in the day was something special.

The bike was brilliant, at least I thought it was but later that year I had my head well and truly turned when I first saw the Kawasaki H2 750. Oh man, what a bike this was, and I was soon making my way down to Smithies to order one, as he was now the Kawasaki dealer. A good three weeks went by until I got the call saying it was ready to collect.

I soon found myself drooling over this purple two stroke triple beast, but needless to say that on getting home I got the silent treatment from my mum again, but what the hell. As you can imagine mum wasn't too pleased at the thought of me getting a bigger bike, but still came out to have a look when I got home, well it more of a glance then a look and was soon going back into the house.

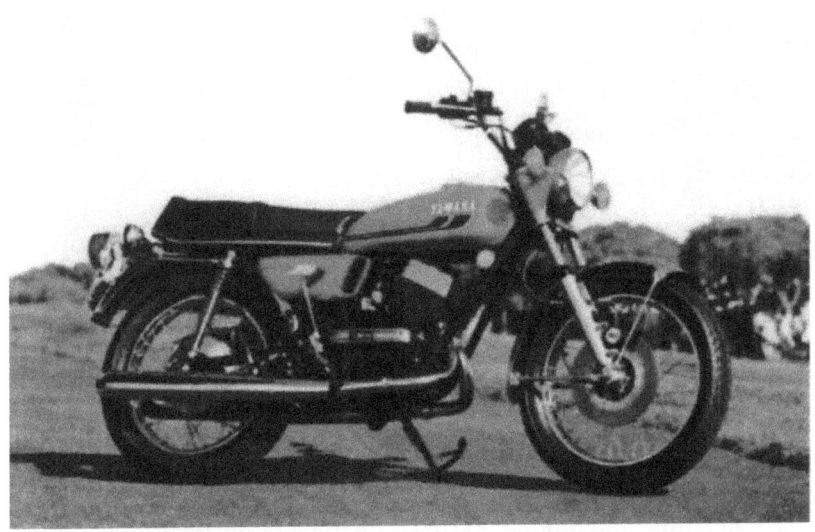

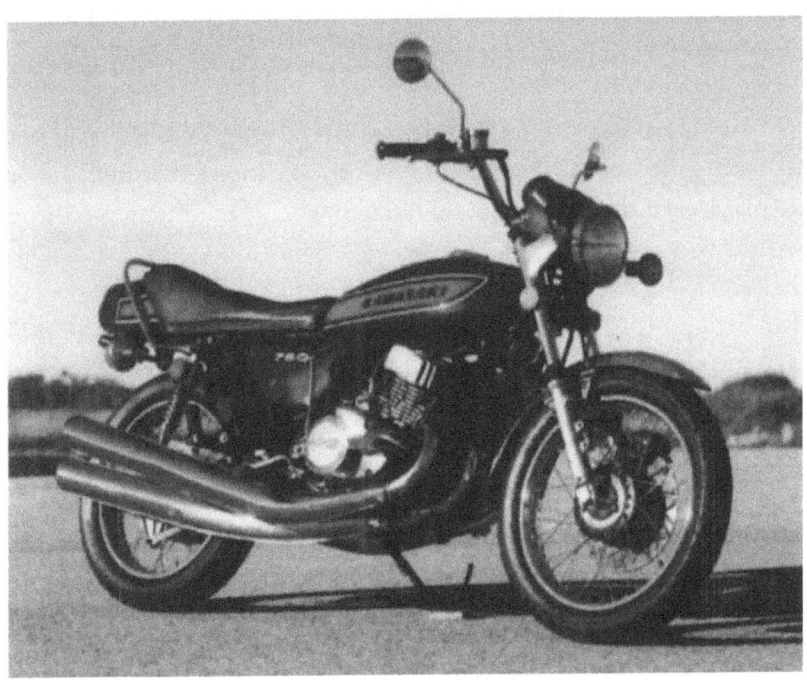

It was now May and Phil asked me if I fancied going to the TT, "Oh yes" I replied, and plans were made that we would go on the 30th of May. I booked the week off work and prepared myself for the trip, it wasn't long before it was D-day, the bike was ready and I was ready, so off I went and headed towards Kirkburton, as I travelled along Peniston Road I approached the junction where you turn left for Kirkburton, I indicated as did the car in front of me, but then the car pulled out to the right then did a sharp left, which put the car going right across my path. Within seconds I had ploughed into the car's passenger door then shot over the handlebars, smashing my right femur on the guttering on the car's roof, then crashing headfirst into the wall on the opposite side of the car.

I was out cold, and it wasn't long before the traffic had started to build up, the police were soon on the scene and tried to get the traffic flowing again, but they didn't seem that interested in my welfare. Luckily for me, in that traffic jam sat Bill Ryan, a nursing officer at Storthes Hall but also a family friend. Bill was soon out of his car and by my side, where he found that I wasn't breathing and quickly started CPR and got me breathing again and then handed me over to the ambulance which had just arrived. I was soon on my way to Huddersfield infirmary, where I was assessed in casualty.

I had multiple breaks in my right femur as well as quite a bad head injury and soon ended up in theatre where I had the bones manipulated back into place, then the leg was put on traction with a Steinmann pin through my knee.

After the opp I was put into a side room on ward 16, as I was a little bit crazy and very loud due to the head injury. I stayed there until I was stable and not with the fairies anymore. It took a while before I came around properly and realised where I was, what had happened and come to terms with being stuck in this bloody bed with my leg on traction. The days dragged on but the highlight of the day was visiting time when I got to see mum and dad, and the lads who always cheered me up, its times like this when you know who your friends are, and I must say that my friends were absolutely brilliant.

As I couldn't or wouldn't keep still, it wasn't long before I was back in theatre having my leg reset, as the bones kept coming out of position. I had this done a further three or four times until everything stayed put and I learnt to keep still.

Life on the ward could be pretty boring, but unlike today's hospitals you didn't have to pay to watch tv, and taking into consideration the length of time I spent there it was a good job really as it would have cost me a fortune. We all had different ways of passing time. If you were a reader like a lot on the ward, you could just lay in your bed and read away to your hearts content, but I've never been much of a reader, so I didn't have that option. A lot of the time it all depended on who else was on the ward or if you got someone in the next bed you could have a laugh with the days went a lot quicker, and not forgetting the nursing staff who could always put a smile on my face.

The days I had physio were always a bonus especially on the days I went to the hydro pool, which meant a trip through the hospital on a trolly, which might not seem like a big deal but when you've been looking at the same walls week after week it was like going on a cruise to me. The other highlight of the day was mealtimes, as there wasn't much more to look forward too. I remember one lunch time as I lay in my bed waiting for the chuck wagon to come, I was starving but hey ho, right on que the trolley rolled onto the ward and I soon sat up in my bed waiting for my dinner. The nurse plopped the tray on my table saying "enjoy nige" as she walked away, but as I took the lid off I was horrified to see what was on the plate, I had ordered some beef stew, carrots, peas and potatoes, what I got was one pea, one slice of carrot, one extremely small potato and one little cube of meat. I wasn't a happy bunny at all, but as luck had it my dad had just walked onto the ward. "Have you seen this?" I asked, is it someone's idea of a joke, "well I ain't laughing" replied dad as he looked down at the plate then shot out the ward saying, "I'll bloody kill him". Apparently, dad had bollocked someone in the kitchen that morning and this was their way of trying to get their own back. Dad knew exactly who was responsible and wasn't putting up with any shit from him. That evening mum and dad came to visit and as dad sat down he asked what my evening meal had been like, "very nice" I replied, "well" said dad "if it ever happens again just let me know and I will bloody have him, it's not your fault I've bollocked him, so if he has anything to say, he can say it to me", I just laid there nodding my head as I could see he was still fuming, "ok Jack, lets forget it now" said mum "lets change the subject", "ummm" replied dad as he sat there sipping a cup of tea.

As I lay in my bed totally pissed off as the weather outside was beautiful, I longed to be out there on my bike going for a blast, some where like Cawthorne bends or the road that goes past Holme moss. But as reality struck home, I knew that the farthest I would be going was a trip to x-ray (if I was lucky, lol). Then out the corner of my eye I noticed a nurse walking towards my bed, "now then Nige, have you had your bowels opened?" she asked, "well" I replied "seeing that you mentioned it, no I haven't", "ok" she replied, then made her way across the ward where she stopped to talk to one of the ward sisters. On her return she was holding a metal bowl which she put down on my locker, then pulled the curtains around as I poured myself a glass of water. "now then Nige, whatever you are wearing on your bottom half take off and roll onto your side" which I did straight away. As I lay there, I thought that this must be some special tablet to have the curtains drawn and go through all this palaver, but boy was I in for a shock. "grit your teeth and it will all be over in a few minutes Nige" and before I had any chance to put my glass of water down it was all over, yep I had just had my first suppository and I wasn't a happy bunny.

"Right then Nige, hold tight for about fifteen minutes and I will be back with the bed pan". Well that must have been the longest 15 minutes of my life before she returned. I soon found myself swinging from the bar above the bed then lowering myself down onto the bloody thing. The rest is history apart from been to messy to write about, but that was one experience I will never forget.

As I lay in my bed the next morning still reeling from the bed incident the ward clerk approached my bed, "you have some post Nige", "Oh good, just pop it down on my locker" which she did then carried on about her business. The first one was a card from my aunty Bet in Birmingham and the second one looked very official, in a brown envelope and printed across the back were the words Gainsborough Council. As I opened it, I could see it was a red one, so I quickly read on. It was from the council whose streetlight I demolished in the accident and they wanted £350 to replace the light, so after a few heated phone calls and a lot of shouting they eventually backed down and wrote the money off. But just when you think it can't get any worse, WRONG.

The ward clerk returned with yet more post, this time it was a letter from the DHSS requesting that I have a medical and he wasn't a happy chappy, "can I take the letter with me?" He asked "sure you can" I replied as he made a swift exit out of the ward and back to his office. I don't know what he had said to them, but I never heard any more apart from a letter cancelling the medical.

The weeks were dragging on and I was still in the same position I was when I was admitted, then into the ward walked Mr Williams, my consultant, who came straight up to my bed and said "we're going to fit you a calliper" "oh, right" I replied, "what will that do?" I asked. He then explained that it was a metal frame that fitted into the heel of my shoe and a ring at the top of my thigh that I sat on, so I could walk without putting any weight on my broken bones, which in the long run would give the femur more time to mend.

That day I was measured up for the calliper and two weeks later it arrived, and I was shown how to put it on and how to walk around on it. Walking on it to start with wasn't easy as it didn't bend, so you had to swing your leg out to the side, but I soon mastered it and was making good progress, when the physio told me that once I had mastered the stairs Mr Williams might let me go home.

The following Monday was doctors rounds and as it got to my turn to be looked at, he stood and flicked through my notes "ummm, and how is he doing with his walking? Especially the stairs?" he asked, "very well indeed" said the physio, "well in that case I can't see any reason why you shouldn't go home today". I was so pleased to be going home, but at the same time a little sad to be leaving all the wonderful staff who had looked after me and so kind. Good old NHS.

I had not been home long before Hugh called up for a coffee and a natter, that evening he came back and walked me up to the pub as I was still very unsteady to say the least. It was good to be getting out again but everything was such hard work especially walking with the bloody calliper on and it was all up hill to the pub, but I wasn't going to be beaten, so it was head down one step at a time. Most evenings were spent in the pub as it was a good excuse to get together with the lads (and lasses) most nights there would be Hugh and his sister Judith, Carol and Mick, Jen, Andrew and Peter, Paul and Janet, Terry, Dave and Mel, and some I can't remember the names of.

George the landlord really looked after us, even though some of the older customers thought we were rowdy, but he wouldn't have a word said against us and started doing hotdogs and burgers as well as a disco every week.

It was a Saturday morning and we had decided to go to Barnsley Kawasaki centre and I had borrowed a 200cc Yam for the journey, but as I had the calliper on I had to hook the end of it onto a nut on the front wheel, happy days I was mobile again. All went well until we got about half way when the calliper slipped off the nut and my heal dug into the tarmac lifting me out of the seat and beading the calliper backwards, but I stopped on and it wasn't until we got to the Kawasaki centre that I discovered what damage I had done to it. On returning home we went straight to my garage where I took the calliper off and it was straightened out so that my parents would be none the wiser.

By now I had got pretty good on the calliper but it was still a pain in the bum not being able to bend it, but Monday was the day I was going to see the consultant, who hopefully would say that it could come off. Well happy days, that's exactly what he said. It was a bit scary at first walking without it as my leg was so skinny and weak and bending the bugger wasn't that easy either.

The time was flying by and my leg was getting stronger and I had just started back to work when Yamaha brought out the new RD 400, OH WOW, what a bike this was and I was soon down at Silvesters to order one. I must say that I wasn't the most popular person in our house when I said what I was getting, but what the hell, I got one anyway. When I picked it up form Silvesters I was buzzing, it was a fast bugger and it handled pretty good, but I was just happy to be on two wheels again. The following weekend mum and dad went to Birmingham to see dads family and Chris and myself had decided to go to see Mez race, but little did I know it was going to be a day that would change my life forever.

It was a lovely Sunday morning when we set off for Caldwell and headed towards Doncaster and Bawtry, where we decided to stop for a coffee in a little café about halfway down the main street. After a quick pitstop we were on our way again and quickly approaching the bridge at Gainsborough. I can't remember how fast I was going but it was no walking pace, lol. When halfway around the last bend before the bridge, my back-tyre burst, I can't remember much apart from my back wheel then started to collapse and by now I was sliding along the rim when the bike mounted the pavement and I got close and personal with a street light and I was out cold.

The usual shit happens next, the cops and the ambulance arrived. The scene was sealed off and I was carted off to Lincoln county hospital where I ended up in intensive care.

The outlook wasn't good, the police were asked to get hold of my parents as soon as they could as they only gave me about three hours to live. They called Huddersfield police station to see if they could track down my parents. Lucky the copper that answered was a family friend who knew that they were in Birmingham and soon got the phone number for dads' sister where they were stopping and told them of the severity of my condition. Dads brother said that he would drive them up to Lincoln as dad was in no state to drive and they were soon on their way.

On arrival at the hospital the specialist told them that it was only a matter of hours and there wasn't a lot he could do apart from try and make me comfortable until the inevitable happened, but sadly there was nothing more he could do. As the hours turned into days then weeks I was still hanging in there, the specialist said to my dad "he must have some fight in him! Because its beyond me how he's still with us". As weeks went by and my condition started to stabilize the decision was made to transfer me back to Huddersfield royal infirmary, where I was soon been wheeled back onto ward 16, where I eventually opened my eyes.

At first I thought I was dreaming so went back to sleep but when I woke again, yep I was still there and to me it only seemed like seconds ago when I was on the bike but as reality started to sink in I got to realise a lot of weeks had passed by since I was last in the land of the living and it wasn't long before I was surrounded by medical professionals.

They ran test after test, I don't think there's a test they didn't do on me. As I lay there totally oblivious to what was going on and trying to make some sense of it all, I was soon in the company of some guy in a white coat who asked me if I could feel anything, "like what?" I asked, "well anything at all" he replied, "no" I said, "I have a slight tingling in my right arm but that's about it".

Just then dad walked onto the ward and asked the specialist what he thought, "well" he replied "Nigel has taken a very serious blow to the head, which has left his right side very weak and his left side is partially paralysed and in my opinion he will not get much of it back, so unfortunately what he has now is about as good as it gets". I just lay there with tears rolling down my face, dad got closer to my bed and stroked my head and said "well lad you have done it good and proper this time" I was speechless. For the next couple of days, I just lay there thing thinking about what had been said and the kind of life I was going to have, not being able to do the things I always took for granted. Even the simple things like getting washed or feeding myself were now things that I couldn't do anymore, and walking was just a dream. Being in this state wasn't the way I wanted to spend the rest of my life, and being the stubborn pig headed twat I am, I decided that I wasn't going to listen to what the specialist had to say, and I was going to prove them all wrong.

As I lay there for hours with my arms on pillows, I wouldn't take me eyes off my fingers willing them to move, and after what seemed like a lifetime I got a little movement in on one finger, and in my world where there was movement there is hope and over the following weeks I continued with my master plan until I could slowly walk my fingers up and down the pillow, but I still had to be washed and fed and all drinks were given to me in a F-ing pink feeder beaker. Meal times got harder as I decided that I wanted to feed myself and devised a way of holding the fork but it was a lot harder getting food on the bloody thing and near on impossible getting it into my mouth without ending up covered in the stuff, as the muscles had wasted and the coordination had a mind of its own, which was usually anywhere but my mouth. Some of the other patients were having bets on whether I would hit my mouth or not, but I persevered and just like a baby I taught myself how to feed myself again and all the other things I couldn't do. It was hard work but giving up wasn't an option so I fought on until I got a lot better at feeding myself, but I still wasn't perfect by any standard, but at least I was getting more in my mouth then on my chest. But little did I know that had been easy against what I had in mind next.

Things don't always go at the speed you want them to, so yet more day's passed by and the days soon turned into weeks, I was getting more and more frustrated with myself and my situation. There wasn't a lot I could do about it; I just had to sit back and bide my time and do the best with what I had got! Which wasn't a great deal. All I seemed to hear was, "no no no Nigel you can't do that, and the faster you get used to the facts the easier it's going to be on you", who were these people and how did they know so bloody much about what I could and couldn't do. I'm not that stupid that I didn't know that a specialist was a specialist for a reason, but hey everyone makes mistakes or doesn't look at the bigger picture every now and then, and just because medical books went against everything I was thinking about doing doesn't mean they were right, and hey I didn't have anything to lose by giving things a try.

It seemed to me that everyone was telling me the same crap, and the more I was told, the more I would rebel and do the exact opposite. In between dreaming about what and how I was going to go about doing the thing I knew I had to do, there was I normal boring life to contend with on the ward. My way of thing was, what they didn't know wouldn't hurt them, so I would pick my times very carefully so no one would get suspicious. That at times I found very hard as my whole world revolved around a single bed and a locker, but no one was going to get in my way as I marched ahead with my master plan.

I was spending more and more time preparing myself for the day I would be able to walk again without crutches or anything else that they would call an aid. I knew the day was fast approaching where I had just got to bite the bullet and get on with it, no matter what the consequences. My head was in a right state, with keeping so many secrets but I couldn't afford to slip up now as my mind was firmly set on what I had to do and when I was going to do it, as that day was getting closer and closer. I WAS ready, that night after lights out I was determined to walk, it didn't matter how far, it was a start, and that night after lights out, I made my move.

So I put plan B into operation, that I was going to get out of this bloody bed and try to get my legs to move, which I was told it just wasn't going to happen. But me being me didn't want to believe this so I hatched a plan to give it a go. After the visitors had gone we always had a last drink before settling down for the night and lights out, then 45 minutes later one of the night staff would come around with her torch making sure we're all settled in and sleeping and right on cue here she was shuffling around the Ward when she got to me I just lay there with my eyes tightly shut until she went back to the nurses station.

Well I thought this is it as I dragged my right leg out from under the sheets followed by my left leg, and there I sat on the edge of the bed, as I hadn't been up for such a long time my head was spinning and I was dizzy as hell.

I sat for a few more minutes until it stopped and then I made my move. I slid out of the bed until my feet were on the floor and just stood there for a bit holding on to the bed, as I looked down at my feet I kept saying to myself "well come on you bastards move!" but nothing was happening, until I managed to slowly slide my right foot forward a couple of inches, but the left one wasn't playing the game and wouldn't move at all so I let go of the bed and put my hands around my knee and moved it manually but as I went to move the right foot again I got a right wobble on and went crashing down knocking my table over on the way and smacking my head on the bottom of the bed and consequently waking all the ward up. The night staff were soon on scene and got me back into bed, where I had my head wound seen to and a bit of a bollocking but I had broad shoulders so it went in on one ear and out the other lol. As I lay there, the nurse ranted on, and I was planning my next move.

The next morning, I was the talk of the ward as well as getting a telling off from the ward manager, and just when you think it can't get any worse, in walked my dad. "what the hell did you think you were doing" he asked, "well just laying there everyday ain't going to get me anywhere is it, no matter what they say, I don't intend on spending the rest of my days in a bed or a wheelchair being fed and washed and given a drink out of that fucking feeder beaker".

Dad just stood there looking at me for a few minutes then said, "well I guess I can't argue with that" as he turns around and walked out muttering "I'm off back to my office". "Umm" I thought "that wasn't that bad" but he could read me like a book and knew that no matter what I was told I was always going to do what I wanted even if that meant doing the exact opposite. The next few nights I was watched like a hawk so I played the game and stopped where I was, that was until it had all blown over and then I tried again, and this time I managed two steps before hitting the deck.

On the 4th or 5th attempt I decided I would try and walk around my bed and thought that if I kept close I could slightly lean on the bed for support and hopefully get further and happy days it worked and I shuffled my way around the bed, getting back in on the opposite side. Now I was totally knackered and soon fell asleep. In the morning I was woken by a nurse for breakfast, who commented on how well I had slept and was none the wiser about my excursion around the bed. After a few more attempts and a lot more falls, my dad was summoned to the ward office where he was told that the decision had been made to discharge me.

Dad asked if that was a good idea "you've seen the state of him", they agreed but said being on the ward wasn't the right place for me as I had proved I wasn't willing to do as I was told and if I was determined to do my own thing I might as well be at home.

Dad didn't totally agree but the next day they came to pick me up, and if I'm being honest I was a mess but I knew that at home there would be more challenges for me to conquer if I was ever to have a half normal life, this was the only way. As we pulled outside the house, I noticed my first obstacle, the steps up to the kitchen door. Oh well I was here now and that was the only way in, so I slid out of the car and slowly made my way up the steps and by the time I had got into the kitchen I was shattered and soon found myself fast asleep on the sofa. When I awoke I was given a cup of coffee by my grandad who was very pleased to see me as he had lent me the money to get the bike and thought it was his fault, but I soon explained that if I had not got the money off of him I would have got it somewhere else and still got the bike which made him feel a bit better.

By the end of the day I was knackered, this being at home wasn't that easy, but I knew I had no choice in the matter and knew that I had to get on with it no matter what. Over the next couple of days things cropped up that I had never even thought about like getting in the shower and getting dressed. The first morning was a killer, I had woken about 7 ish, slowly made my way into the bathroom where I got washed and shaved, it was a bit like the chainsaw massacre, but I got there eventually. I now had to get dressed.

Getting my jeans on wasn't that hard but the T-shirt was a different matter and after a good couple of hours there was only the shoes left. Well I was like a one year old trying to do the laces up, the coordination was still pretty naff so doing the laces was a work of art which ended up in a knotty mess but that's the best I could do for now, and after a good two and a half hours I made my way downstairs.

As I spent weeks doing various things to try and improve the strength and coordination in what was still a very knackered body. Some days it seemed like I was fighting a losing battle and thoughts were the days where I had to pick myself up and push on regardless.

I would spend hours sat on a chair in my bedroom practising walking my fingers up the bedroom walls as well as trying to pick things up with my fingers and thumb, and anything else that would help in my fitness regime, eating was still a big problem that I struggled with, so this was something I spent a lot of time practising, and fastening shirt buttons up was a nightmare especially when it came to the right side cuff with my left hand (it was and still is impossible). I would cheat a little and fasten my cuffs first then squeeze my hands down the shirt sleeves. Tying my shoelaces was a big headache which could take up to an hour in the early day.

But regardless of anyone or anything I carried on regardless, coz if I was ever going to conquer this thing I was left with, there was no going back, just forward.

Everything just took forever, or that's how it seemed to me, but I found a part of me that I didn't know existed, that was patient and I realised early on that I would need a lot if I was to get anywhere, but its amazing what you can achieve if you want it hard enough and your willing to push yourself to the edge and then that little bit further, no matter what the doctors and physios and specialists tell you, if you have faith in yourself and what you believe in, you can achieve a lot more than the medical books would have you believe.

So it was head down and keep on trying, there were lots of days where I could have quite easily given in especially when there was something that I found really hard to do like walking without looking like I was pissed, but that wasn't going to happen for a long time and it's something I just had to come to terms with. Each day was a battle which brought its own problems, and each problem was a battle which had to be sorted out before I could move on to the next stage when it all started again. Things like getting showered and dried seemed to take forever and I was still struggling with getting dressed. When it came to getting shaved, well what can I say it was a blood bath as my coordination was still pretty crap, I only shaved when I had to, which luckily wasn't that often. Then there was the shoelaces which I still struggled with big time but I always managed to do it, no matter how long it would take me, or what a knotty mess I got them in eventually I would get there, even though it always took forever.

The days were long but there was always something to do or a body part to work on which all rolled together towards my end goal. At times it seemed like everything I wanted to do, there was someone there saying, "no Nige, you'll never be able to do that" or "forget it Nige and do it another way". There was no room for compromise or short cuts not in my master plan. The things that I found hard or impossible to do I would do over and over until I got better at it, and if I'm being honest the only thing that I really never mastered was the buttons on my shirt cuffs, which was and still is far to F-ing fiddly to get my head around. Most things that I came up against and after giving them a lot of thought I could get the better of, but the things that were out of my control like my limp, and in the early days my slurred speech would really drive me mad, but it was always head down and best foot forward and who knows what I'm going to achieve, but I was damn sure that I was going to achieve a hell of a lot more in my life then I was told I could only dream of, coz sometimes being pig headed and stubborn can get you a hell of a long way.

Outwardly everyone thought I was coping but that was far from the truth, yes, I was getting on with my life and still making progress, but I was so frustrated as it just wasn't happening fast enough for me. Even though I had good support from family and friends, I couldn't bring myself to tell anyone how I was really feeling, which looking back made things far worse for myself. At the time I didn't want to let anyone know how much I was struggling with the state of my mental health and how much I longed to be normal again, this mental battle that was going on in my head was harder to beat than any broken bones.

Eventually progress picked up and for the first time I knew I had a goal in sight, when that would be I didn't know, good job really as I'm now 62 and still not quite there but hey I had come this far and the bastard ain't going to beat me now.

The days came and went but my battle for fitness was nonstop, but sadly there were always problems especially with my left leg, and I always seemed to be in hospital having surgery on the damn thing and each time it took longer to recover.

There were days when I could have gladly laid down and died but that was admitting defeat, and it would have been a bit messy, how the hell can you overdose when you struggle to get food in your mouth. Thanks to the support I had from everyone I would always bounce back but the whole situation was driving me mad and very short tempered to the point where I didn't like myself anymore. Everything was much harder than I imagined and trying to get the bend in my knee to 45 degrees was just not happening. Getting on the exercise bike was a work of art as I had to have the seat a lot higher to compensate for the lack of bend in the knee but I was getting nowhere fast, so one night as I tried to pedal all the way around as usual when it got near the top it wouldn't go any further so I stood up on the pedals and gritted my teeth then forced my bum downwards into the saddle, the pain was unbearable but hey the knee was bent and I slowly managed to get the pedals all the way around.

As I got off the bike and staggered to the bathroom, I was like bambi on ice, but what the hell, I had done it and hopefully without doing anymore damage. I sat in the bathroom for a while until I had stopped shaking, then got washed, which was still a battle, then made my way downstairs very slowly on my bum. As I wobbled into the lounge where dad was sat reading the paper "what the hell have you been up to?" he asked, "you don't want to know" I replied as I slithered into a chair.

I then went through a stage where everything got me down, and I couldn't be bothered trying anymore and just stopped everything, exercising, dieting and going out was a pain, I really didn't want to be me anymore. It was around this time one evening when we had visitors at home and no matter who it was, I knew what they were going to say, things like: you cant tell you limp (well you noticed), I can see your arms no better (umm just what I wanted to hear) and the one that really pissed me off was, do you manage to get out much? (no, they lock me in my room when they go to work, as I'm such a liability) but I would resist replying as I didn't want to offend. Mum would bring in the mugs of tea and I could hear whispers of, well doesn't he hold his mug funny, Audrey? I don't think he will get over this one, they should have kept him in hospital, with his problems he isn't going to have much of a life. I'm not deaf you know, I blurted out, and then got the look from my dad so I shut up.

Just when you think it cant get any worse I heard someone say, you've got your hands full there Audrey, that's one young man you're going to be stuck with for a very long time, but mum wasn't having any of it and soon put her in her place. I'd just decided to go to the loo when someone said, you'll have to be his carer Audrey and he will need a specially adapted room, and what about when you want to go out, how long can you leave him for? (I was speechless). Everyone was a fucking doctor all of a sudden, who were these people anyway, with their big ideas and bigger mouths, I'd heard so much so I went upstairs to my room and got on the exercise bike and pedalled and pedalled and pedalled, then did some sit ups and squats against the wall, then back on the bike and did it all again. As for the visitors they might have been self-opinionated pricks, but it gave me the reality check that I needed to get myself back on track and push forward.

Over the following weeks I really got my mojo back and my expectations were still very high, because if I didn't set the bar high I couldn't see much was going to change and in my head that was totally unacceptable. I would still sit and practise picking pennies up with my fingers and also walking my fingers up the wall, in fact I would do anything I could that helped me get back the strength and coordination in my arms and legs. But even though I was making good progress I still struggled with eating, getting that fork into my mouth wasn't always easy, especially when I thought people were looking, as I was so self-conscious and a little embarrassed.

As well as my wish to overcome the accident it gave me the incentive to lose weight, as well as get as fit as I possibly could. The exercise bike came out in the bedroom and it was back to basics with my food and drink, and every night I went through an exercise program before getting into bed. I would go on the bike, I would do sit ups, and sit on the edge of the bed and walk my fingers up the wall as I was struggling to get the left one higher than my shoulder. The thing that really got me was trying to improve the coordination in my fingers, this was really hard. I would spread out pennies and two pennies on the top of my dressing table then try picking them up with different fingers and my thumb working across to my little finger. It sounds easy but when you can't do it no matter how hard you try, it gets very frustrating, but hey, I had plenty of time to practise and try and master the dreaded penny challenge.

By now I had lost quite a lot of weight and was totally obsessed with getting fitter, but tended to keep what I was doing to myself and would do most things in my bedroom or in the garage, and very slowly it all kind of started to fall into place, my arms were getting stronger and getting more use in them, my legs were also responding very well and the weight was still coming off. Even though my legs were getting stronger I had one leg shorter than the other so I couldn't do a lot about the limp the I had but that was the least of my problems on the grand scheme of things, as walking any distance was a killer and I still struggled feeding myself, but I was 100% better than I was when I came out of hospital.

By now a good eight months had passed since I had come home and in my eyes I had not achieved what I wanted to achieve, but as far as the specialists were concerned I was doing more than they had hoped for, but being my own critic was what kept me going, but without the backup that I had from my family and especially my friends I guess I could have easily given in.

On one particular visit to the hospital I asked if I could go the following week to a doctors seminar where they could discuss my case and some of the operations that I had gone through, and it wasn't long before I found myself examined by consultants from all over, who were very impressed by my achievements and the things I had done to get where I was at the present. As it was now time for me to try getting back to work I would need transport, but with all that I had been through I dare not mention getting a motorbike as I think mum and dad would have gone loopy, and my body couldn't take any more knocks. So, I started learning to drive dad's car, it was all right but not as exciting as the bike but this time I had no option, it was either the car or the bus!

As I slowly got back into the routine of going to work and all that it entailed, I soon found myself looking at the ladies instead of the bikes and found out just what I had been missing out on.

There was one good looker that worked in the kitchen office who had really caught my eye and I soon found myself stuttering and stammering as I tried to ask her out on a date at the weekend.

I was very surprised when she said that she would love to, that weekend we went to the clothiers at Shelley for a drink and found that we really got on well, and just look at what I had been missing out on all this time. Over the next few months, we saw a lot of each other, and it got really serious, to the point where I asked her to marry me, and happy days she said yes.

The wedding was planned, and we had also bought a house in Highburton by the time the big day arrived, and we walked down the aisle. The wedding was held at the main church in Huddersfield and the service was done by a cannon knox and after the service we had the reception at a place in Almondbury and in the evening we also had a disco there. Life was good and everything was going fine, I had a new wife, a good job and a sort of new car and hadn't had any trouble with my health for quite a number of months, so what could go wrong? I had everything I wanted.

After a couple of years, we decided to move closer to work to cut the traveling out and house prices had gone up, so we were going to make a tidy profit out of the sale of our house. We soon found a house in Crosland moor which was only two minutes from work and moved in, but by now we had started to drift apart, and it wasn't long before she moved out and we started divorce proceedings. I had just started a new job in a new market supermarket in Huddersfield which meant we didn't work together anymore, which I guess was a good thing. After a few months I started dating someone id met at work and everything was fine and we decided to move to Cleethorpes for a fresh start as that was where she came from.

Life in Cleethorpes was pretty good, I also got a job working in the kitchen at RAF North Coates. The camp was in the middle of nowhere, about twenty-two miles from Cleethorpes. Just as I got the job my car gave in on me and I needed transport asap so I rented a small motorbike from a place just around the corner from where I lived, but it was winter and bloody cold on a bike especially when I was on early shift, but needs must as there wasn't any other options open to me, the job was good and I was there about a year or so until the base closed down. At the same time as losing my job my left knee started to play up again and soon found myself going back to Huddersfield to see the consultant who recommended further surgery as soon as there was an available bed. Within a day or so I was back on the ward preparing myself for yet more surgery. On been discharged I went back to Cleethorpes and slowly got back to normal but things were not good and soon found myself getting divorced and moving into a house in Grimsby on my own, but that year I ended up going back for yet more surgery on my very unstable left knee. After this operation, things were really good and I kind of forgot about my left knee and moved house again into a flat on the seafront in Cleethorpes were I had only been about two weeks when I got a job as a chef in a residential home. I had been there for about two months when the owner asked if I fancied moving into the empty room on the top floor, umm how much? I asked, you can have it rent free Nige, he replied. I agreed and the following week I moved in.

I was there a good three years without any problems and then I started to get a lot of pain in my left knee again, so it was back to Huddersfield where I had more work done. I came around from the anaesthesia, I realised that I had a huge pot on which went from my hip to my toes, bugger, I would have to drag this bloody thing around with me for weeks, which really pissed me off. When I got out of the hospital I went back to my dads for a few days and then decided I would go back to Cleethorpes, and how the hell do you intend getting back he asked, well I'll drive back obviously I replied, what with that bloody pot on! Yes I muttered, I'll be fine. Later on that day I packed up my stuff and slid into my car where I carefully lifted the leg onto the clutch, as I couldn't bend the leg when I wanted to change gear I had to move my leg up and down from the hip. It wasn't easy but it got me to the motorway where I thought that once I was in top gear it would be a piece of cake, little did I know what lay in front of me.

As I headed up the M62 with my foot resting to the left of the clutch everything was fine, I couldn't see what all the fuss was about and carried on without any problems until I got about eight miles from Grimsby and by now it was getting really busy with the tea time traffic, as you get to the of the motorway there are three big roundabouts that I had totally forgotten about and I was in the middle of a long line of traffic all slowing down for the first roundabout.

I went to change gear, but my left leg was numb and the pot was wedged down the side of the clutch, what the fuck was I going to do now! Well there was just enough room between the lines of cars for one mini metro so I pulled out and made my way between the lines of cars until I got to the roundabout where I said a quick prayer and barged my way around. Well that was one out of the way, only two to go. The other drivers were honking their horns and waving their arms, but I just waved back and carried on regardless. I manoeuvred my way around the second roundabout like someone on the dodgems and by the time I got to the last one I had a bit of life back in my leg so I lifted it onto the clutch and slowly made my way around it, and by the time I got back to Cleethorpes I was knackered but hey I had done it and got back in one piece.

I hobbled into the lounge were I was met by Ann the matron who was very surprised to see me and even more surprised to learn how I had got back and just shook her head and said "only you". I spent the rest of the day chilling out and catching up on the gossip until Ann asked me if I would like to go to one of the empty downstairs rooms for a few weeks to stop me having to climb all the stairs to my room. Good idea I said and that's just what I did until the pot came off.

As soon as I was able, I started going back to Spartana (which was a gym not far from work) the owner John Farnham taught me loads and the more

I got to know the more I wanted to know and soon found myself in the position where I would rather be in the gym than at work but I needed the money so I just got on with it. By now I was back on my feet and back working when I started going out with one of the care assistants and life was back on track and eventually we got married (yep I love wedding cake) but it wasn't long after that my leg started playing up again and started swelling up and was extremely painful to bend but unfortunately I couldn't get in to see the specialist in Huddersfield for a couple of weeks so I just had to put up with it, but as I stumbled around Cleethorpes one day I thought of an idea which I thought would help.

By now I had tried most things to stop me bending my leg but nothing worked, so I came up with the idea of building a cage around it out of some old meccano that I had seen for sale in a charity shop and that's just what I did. I stuck the cage to my leg with Elastoplast and initially it worked really well, but one day as I was walking through Cleethorpes I kept hearing a tinkling sound behind me and as I turned around, there scattered all over the pavement was my meccano, oh well it was a good idea at the time. Luckily it wasn't long before I was back in Huddersfield and having yet MORE surgery to put things right but this time I got an infection.

I got an infection in the wound and only a day after been kicked out I ended up back on the ward been pumped full of antibiotics and soon made a full recovery. On returning to Cleethorpes it wasn't long before we moved into a house near the seafront and life got back to normal.

That year the new disability law came in and I ended up at Grimsby college been interviewed by Ann and Jenna from the personnel department who told me they were looking for someone with a disability that was also into fitness and I fitted the bill completely. Initially it was only for twelve weeks but they would also put me through my qualifications as well as giving me work I experience. Well I jumped at such a chance and the following week started at Bargate Fitness Suite. At the end of the twelve weeks I was offered a job but there wasn't enough hours to make it viable and that's when mike (who worked in the gym) gave me some of his hours so I could take the job.

The first couple of years flew by, I was now working full time and also sitting for more qualifications, and this time they were for teaching clients with disabilities and by the end of that year I had got my YMCA qualification in teaching disabled clients, which was on top of my OCR qualifications and then I was told that I had been awarded the student of the year award, I was pleased, the only thing that I got at school was a smack around the head!!

A short time after this I found out I had been put forward for a star award which is given to people who have achieved a lot in their lives and also given a lot back.

It wasn't long before I was off to Leeds for the reginal finals and I am pleased to say that I won my category which also put me into the national finals in London and that year myself, Lee and Joe were off to the big event and anybody who was anything in education or fitness was there and they started to call out the winning names, my heart was in my mouth, it started with the runners up first then working their way up to the finalists and by now there were only first and second place left to call out and I guessed I hadn't made it by this point, when over the loudspeaker I heard "and second place is Nigel Bolton" and I slowly made my way onto the stage to accept my award and the cheque that went with it.

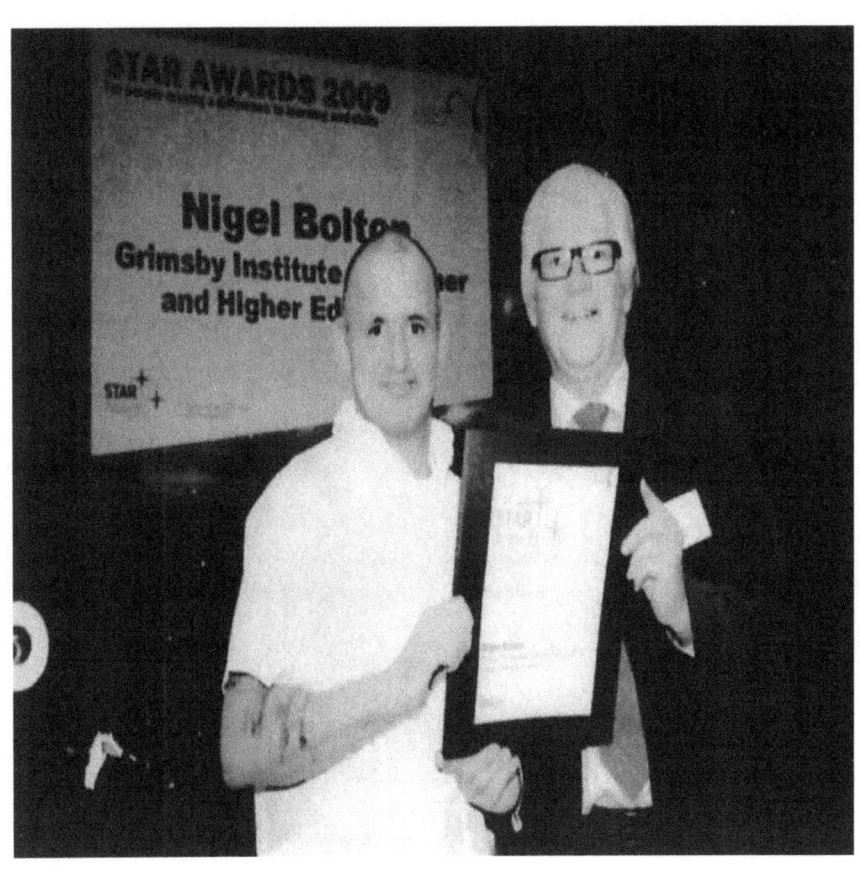

Highly Commended in the category of
Support role

Nigel Bolton
Grimsby Institute of
Further and Higher Education

Sponsored by UNISON

Nominated in the category of
Support role

Nigel Bolton
Bargate Fitness Suite, Grimsby Institute of
Further and Higher Education

Sponsored by UNISON

After the awards, my mum got breast cancer and after a short illness. She died in hospital. It was a big blow to all my family especially my dad who didn't cope very well at all. After the funeral I threw myself into my work as that was my way of dealing with it, on Monday morning shortly after opening up, in walked Dave Moore, Dave was am ex-pro footballer who was now in physio at Grimsby town FC as well as being a first class guy. "Morning Dave, have a good weekend" "I had a brilliant weekend Nige, I went to wales and ran up Snowdon", "Oh wow, well done" I replied, but all that day I couldn't get Snowdon out of my mind.

That night when I got home the house was in darkness and the door was locked which I found pretty strange and when I got in the lounge there was a note on the coffee table which I picked up and started reading, the note said that she had gone and not to look for her as she was starting a new life. Within a week I had worked out where she was, she had moved in with her driving instructor somewhere out of town, so after the initial shock of it all I got on with my life and bought an MX5 sports car and went on holiday to Greece, through it all my work mates were brilliant and involved me in everything and kept me thinking positively. It wasn't long before I started dating again and putting my life back in order again and that's when I started thinking about Snowdon again and came up with the idea of doing a sponsored climb up Snowdon with all the money going to the Hospice, but many people had been up Snowdon so I had to make it special so it stood out and that's when I decided to do it all on crutches.

At the end of the day my legs were knackered anyway so I wouldn't be able to walk up there normally. I got some crutches and started training but it wasn't to long before the local paper ran a story on me followed by a spot-on look north and BBC radio, but the publicity gave the sponsors money a great boost. Also, on board with me was Mike Burton, Sue Tyrell and a local businessman Harp, Mike would be my eyes planning the route on the way up. Sue was there in case I pulled a muscle or strained something, and Harp, he just wanted to come along. The training went well, and everything was in place for the big day. Claire who worked on reception was in charge of the sponsor money and keeping record of who had sponsored what, the day before we went to Wales she had a tally up and as I walked through reception she said "no pressure Nige, I've just counted up the sponsor money, if you do it its around £2,500 so you've got to do it now" "oh wow" I said as I walked away with a smile on my face, and as far as I was concerned if I had to get on my hands and knees and dragged myself to the top I was going to do it.

As the day got nearer, the college where I worked told me that they would pay for the hotel accommodation and let us have a college car to get there and back in and they were paying for the petrol, and that week we set off for wales.

On arriving we booked in and decided to have a look around but soon ended up in a pub and then another one and then ... before we knew where we where it was silly o'clock as we rolled back to the hotel and got some much needed sleep. As we were setting off early the hotel had arranged a special breakfast to be done for us and as we walked into the dining room we were met with a huge buffet style breakfast just for us, so we all dug in and stoked our boilers for the climb ahead. After a short drive we were at the bottom of the mountain and ready for off, Mike smiled and said "well mate it's up to you now", I nodded and we were off. The first part of the climb wasn't that bad, well once I had got the crutches to the right height and then it was head down and just get on with it. The higher we went the steeper it got and a lot harder on my shoulders, by the time we had got halfway the skin under my arms had rubbed off and was bleeding, but every time I stopped for water and the odd protein bar, Mike would pass me the Vaseline which I would slap on. We climbed and climbed but the top just disappeared into the clouds. "Hell, Mike it's getting further away" I muttered, Mike just laughed and said "it was your idea" which I couldn't argue with and marched on. The top was now getting closer but still seemed to be miles away but eventually we were nearly there. "Come on Nige" shouted Mike "your nearly there", as I dragged my very weary butt to the top.

Well I was here, the top of Snowdon (happy days). Under my arms were a right mess and my shoulders and arms just hung there, but what the hell it was over, and it had only taken four and a quarter hours and after a short rest we made our way down, but this time on the train. After a long soak and a sleep, we went out on the town again to celebrate our victory and the next morning we made our way home. Once all the sponsor money was in, the bank had given me one of those big cheques and a representative from the hospice came to the college along with the Grimsby evening telegraph photographer and I handed over the cheque. For a few weeks after people were still talking about that man from Cleethorpes that went up Snowdon on crutches, but the support that I had got from Mike, Sue, Harp and the Grimsby Institute was tremendous, and not forgetting all the kind people that sponsored me.

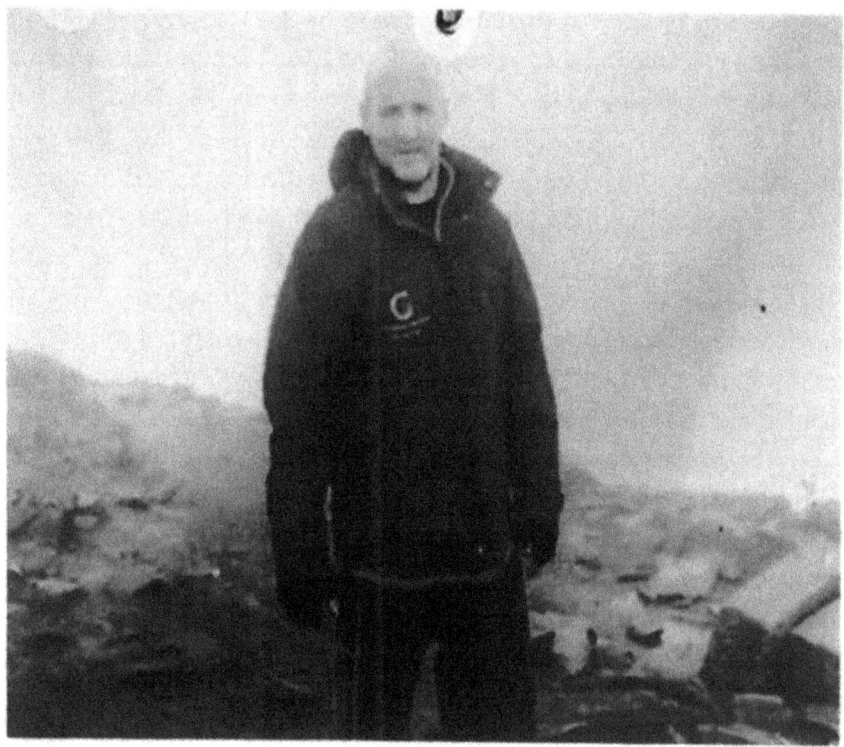

SNOWDON

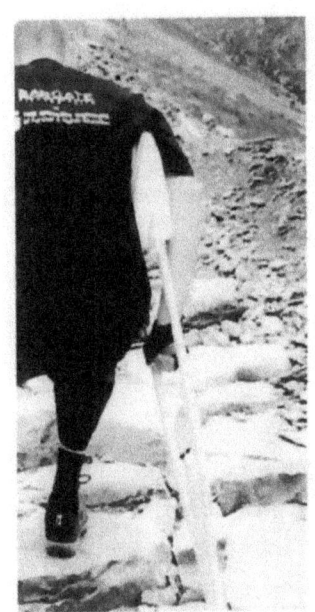
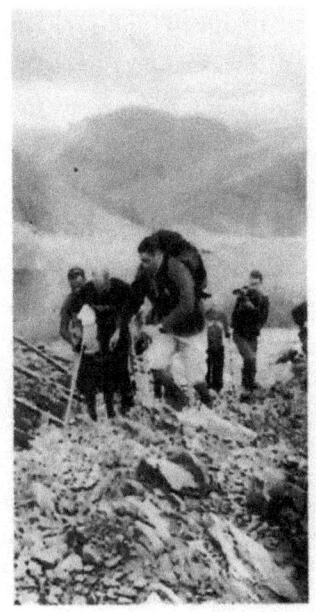
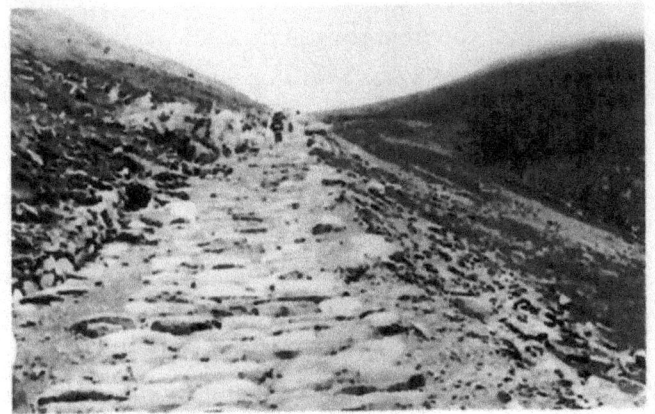

Shortly after the climb I was getting ready for work and just about to go down stairs when I slipped and went flying down the steps at a very fast rate, landing on my left leg and bending it further back then it had been for a lot of years. The pain was off the scales as I lay there for a few minutes composing myself, then I dragged my body up to the phone and called the doctor whose surgery was just around the corner, the receptionist told me that if I wanted to see the doctor I would have to go in! After I went through it again, she then said I could have a home visit, but she didn't know what time it would be. Luckily just then my ex-wives son walked through in and drove me to the hospital. I had an x-ray, I was examined by a consultant that told me my knee would need replacing but I was too young so I should go home and rest it until the swelling goes down and he would see me again in six months. Not a lot of good to me as I couldn't afford not to work and just hang about for six months, so the next day me and my crutches made our way into the gym where I was met by Joe Wood, the boss, who told me to go into the gym and sit on a chair and just supervise, and that's just what I did until later on that morning Dave Moore popped in and was quite surprised to see the state I was in. "And what have you been up to" he asked, so I told him what I had done and what the doctor at the hospital had said.

He wasn't very impressed at all and soon got onto his knees to have a closer look at my knee. "Oh wow, that's very swollen and there's very little movement, you need that seeing to ASAP, in my opinion" then he walked out of the gym saying he would be back later in the day. About two hours later he returned saying he had had a word with Frank the football surgeon and he said he will see you tomorrow in his clinic, and that's just what he did and the following week I was admitted and given a new knee.

After the operation, my knee was very sore and painful, but I had been through a lot worse, so I just got on with it. It wasn't long before the physio had me out of bed and walking about on crutches, and as soon as I could do the stairs, I was sent home. Being at home was very hard work as my wife had just done a runner and doing everything was very hard, if I made a coffee, I then had to get it from the kitchen to my room, it was not easy when you have a crutch in each hand, so I would slide the mug along the worktop as far as I could then put it onto the floor, take two steps forward then move the mud again, I would repeat this until I got to my chair. I did the same thing with my food just sliding the plate across the carpet with my crutch, I did this for weeks and never spilt a drop of coffee or lost any food.

During my time at home I was doing a lot of my own physio, but three times a week I would go to the gym and be sorted out by Dave as the college were paying him to get me back to full fitness and back to work. After a few months I returned to my job. This being at home was alright but there's only so much Jeremy Kyle and Trisha you can take in a day and be back at work was where I wanted to be and soon got back into the routine. I had been seeing a lady from Scunthorpe a couple of times and had arranged to go out again at the weekend but on the Friday lunch she called me at work, she said she couldn't go out with me at the weekend as she had been talking to her husband and they were going to give the marriage another go, "well I hope it works out for you and I hope you are both very happy" I replied, "Don't put the phone down Nige, my husband wants to talk to you", I found this very strange but went along with it and he was soon chatting away. "Is there a point to this conversation" I asked, "well Nige I know you and my wife got along very well and was just wondering if all three of us could get together and _____". "NO NO NO never mate, I wouldn't even share my last rolo with you, never mind what your wanting, you perv" I then hung up and carried on with my day. (I know I like it, but sharing it, NEVER).

Each time I had surgery on my legs I would end up with more scar tissue which meant bending it just got harder and harder, I remember one night in particular when I got into bed after having a naff day with pains in my legs, it started with just spasms in both legs which was very rare as it was usually one leg or the other. I was so tired and just wanted to sleep but the spasms were relentless to the point where it nearly pushed me over the edge and when it got around to 2:45 I was on autopilot and nothing was functioning properly and it all got too much, I grabbed a bottle of Diazepam and poured the lot into my mouth and just sat on the bed crunching away and trying to swallow them but they wouldn't go down.

I must've looked like a right mess with a mouth full of pills and puffy red eyes, but at the time I would've given anything to sleep. What the hell are you doing, I said to myself, if you swallow the pills there is no turning back, so I dragged myself to the bathroom and stuck my fingers down my throat, spitting out the ones I had swallowed as well as the ones in my mouth.

The next day was a fresh start and I never told anyone about the pills, that's until now, and I continued my battle with my disability but it seemed like two steps forward and four steps back but I had no alternative other than going forward, as giving in or settling for second best just wasn't good enough.

As the weeks passed by I soon got back to my old self and started dating again and this time it was a lady from a village near Crowle and as time passed by we moved back to Cleethorpes and started a new life there. After about five years and eight house moves we were moving again into a house right in the middle of Cleethorpes, that's where I ended up back on crutches again and then was admitted to Grimsby Princess Diana Hospital, where I had the false knee taken out and a new one put in. I think I was only in hospital for about four days until I was sent home to recuperate and get mobile again where I put myself through a daily exercise routine as well as lots of walking up and down the street on my crutches and after lots of hours of hard work I was walking unaided again. But I still struggled with the stairs and getting in and out of the bath was virtually impossible so I went to see if there was anything the council could do to help as I had been on their list for a number of years.

Over the next few years, I seemed to spend more time at the hospital than anywhere else, but I couldn't be broken. The more I was told not to do something the more determined I was to do it, no matter what the consequences. It goes without saying that I nearly always got myself into a shed load of trouble, but I just took the tellings off and bollockings and carried on regardless. Yep, if I wanted to do something, I would do it. I guess it was the stubborn pig headedness that kept me going.

I did have my bad days and there were lots of them, but I would always pick myself up and carry on, I struggled a lot with criticism and I still do. I can't stand someone trying to tell me what I should be doing when really, they should shut their big gobs as they haven't a Fucking clue what their talking about. I didn't like that I had a limp as that was one thing, I couldn't do anything about apart from cutting my other leg down to size but that was a bit drastic even for me. People can be so cruel with their little comments and looks, and that got worse the older I got to a certain extent and came to a head when I first joined a dating site after my first divorce. I would start talking to someone on a regular basis and it wasn't long before they would ask if I had all my own teeth and hair, I just laughed it off and said "of course, why? haven't you?" but I knew that before we met I had to mention the limp, sometimes they would just laugh it off and say "so what" but in a lot of cases they would ask how bad a limp and will it get better or how noticeable is it and in a lot of cases they would just say "I don't think I'll bother" and put the phone down, this I found very hurtful even though my friends would tell me that they aren't worth bothering with but it didn't make it any easier finding someone, but hey I kept looking, out of all the twats there must be some nice ones out there. It was just a case of finding one, but I wasn't going to be beat and carried on with my quest.

The nice ones were really nice, and I think one point I just liked going out with someone different every week. I could always tell the ones who were just out for a free night, and there were plenty, but I also met some very nice people, some who are still friends to this day.

I soon found myself in the council offices enquiring about bungalows, only to be told that I wasn't a priority so it would be a long wait, I then explained that I struggled with the stairs and getting in and out of the bath was near impossible for me. The lady then told me that I would have to be assessed by one of their community physios first before I could get re-banded. Three weeks later I was visited by a physio who could see the problems I had with the stairs and the bath and arranged for me to have a bath lift and she could also see the problem with the stairs and said she would submit her report. Two weeks after her visit I received a letter from the council telling me that I had been re-banded which meant I could now look for a bungalow and it wasn't long before one came up on their website and I soon had my name down for it. The bungalow was in Ulceby which is just down the road from Wootton where John and Anne lived, who are the brother and sister-in-law of the lady I was living with at the time. It wasn't long before I got to view it, it had two bedrooms, a bathroom, a big lounge and kitchen, outside there was gardens front and back with plenty of room for a workshop. Luckily, I was on top of the list to view it so I got first refusal but there was no way I was going to let this one pass me by.

That month we moved in and life out in the sticks was just the job. There was a co-op, a pub, a chippy and Barton upon Humber was only a short drive away and Cleethorpes was about twenty minutes, so it wasn't that isolated. We moved in just before Christmas and soon had the trimmings up and for a change everything seemed to be going according to plan (for a change).

The next year I ended up back in hospital having further surgery, this time on my right knee, which I also had to have replaced, the day after the operation I was sent home, where I sat catching up with my post, and in that post was a letter from the DWP who had wrote to tell me they were taking my mobility car off me, which came as a shock as I needed it for getting around as I cant walk that far at all, but what really pissed me off was when I got awarded it. I had it awarded for life, but now that PIP had come into force the government just moved the goal posts to suit themselves no matter what effect it has on the individual in question.

I wasn't going to take this lying down and soon had myself down at the local MP's office who was Mr M Vickers and a conservative. The same people who had brought PIP in, but he didn't agree with it at all and helped me fight my case, and after a great deal of form filling and medicals they backed down and reinstalled my mobility. As things settled down and I got back on with my life, I started getting a lot of pain in my right hip and soon found myself going back to the docs for some advice.

On returning home my partner had her bags packed and told me she was leaving. Well she had spent all my inheritance, so I guess it was time to find a new bank account to milk, and within the hour her son pulled up outside and she was gone. I soon sorted myself out and life wasn't that bad, I still had the same amount of money coming in with one less to keep, and I soon got my bank balance built up again. Been on my own wasn't that bad really, I started dating again and spent a lot of time at John and Anne's, I know that John was her brother but he didn't get involved or take sides, and as a mate he is brilliant. In the first few months I went out with quite a few from all over Lincolnshire, some were very nice, some not! But I had yet to meet someone that really floats my boat and that I really wanted to be with. I kept on looking and then I met a lady from Hull who was nice and we got on, but that sparkle wasn't there, as nice as she was I felt like there was something missing, but then I started to doubt myself, what was I looking for anyway? Who the hell knows, I certainly didn't. I thought I would have some time on my own, so I bought a 1998 Yamaha DT 125 R that had been stood in someone's garden for years and needed a complete renovation. But on stripping it down I discovered that the engine needed a lot of work and that's when John told me about the new Lifan engine that was available online and for less than £300, so I ordered one and as I waited for delivery I stripped the rest of the bike down and took the frame and swinging arm to be powder coated.

A week later I went to Grimsby to pick them up and was very pleased with what I saw, the frame and swinging arm was a sparkly navy blue and looked brilliant, so it was back to Ulceby and start putting it back together.

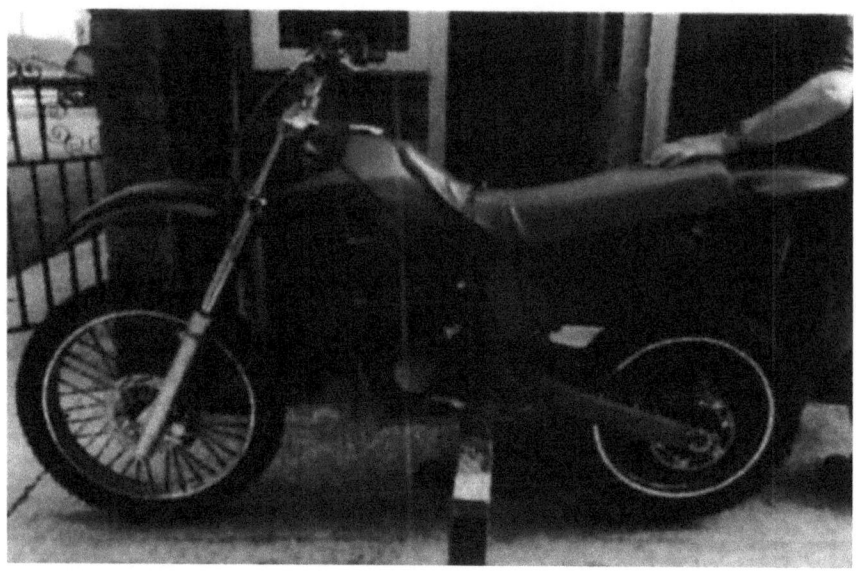

It was a bigger job then I had imagined so I had to take it to the maestro mechanic and good friend John Chafer, who soon had it on the road to recovery. In between helping john with the bike I dated a few more, but there wasn't ever that spark, but I kept on looking until the day I spoke to a lady who lived in Goole who sounded very nice, but me being me, thought that Goole was too far to travel and told her I was very sorry. I spent the next few months on my own but couldn't get her out of my head, so one evening I messaged her and apologised for being a dick and could I take her out, but I would understand if she didn't want to bother, but luckily for me she gave me a second chance and we arranged to meet that weekend.

The weekend soon came around and I was off to Goole to meet Linda, and as I sat in the car waiting, every female with blonde hair walked past my car, and I was so glad they walked past. I got a text from Linda saying she had just left the hairdressers and would only be a few minutes, I sat looking out of the car window and five minutes later there was a blonde-haired lady walking towards the car. Oh wow, if your Linda I'm in heaven I thought as she got closer (and she had thigh length boots on) so hoping that I had the right person I got out of the car clutching a bunch of red roses I walked towards her.

Happy days, it was Linda and after the initial introductions we went to a pub in Snaith for lunch where we sat, chatted and got to know a bit more about each other, by the end of the date we had arranged to meet again and I couldn't wait. We really hit it off from that first date and I was soon going back and forth to Goole so I could be with her on her days off I would go to pick her up and bring her over to Ulceby where I was living, it was during one of those visits when one evening I blurted out "Will you marry me?", she said she would and we were soon making plans for our wedding. As we had both been married before it was going to be at Cleethorpes registry office and I asked John if he and his wife Anne would be our witnesses, and on the 18th of November at 10am we got married and afterwards we went to the Foreshores at Hessel. We started married life living in my bungalow at Ulceby but soon decided to move to Goole, after a frantic search for somewhere to live we found a house on Chiltern Rd and just after Christmas we moved in. We were not very settled there and luckily someone who Linda knew told her that there was a flat coming up in the same block that she had moved out of and luckily we got it and were soon moving in.

The flat was lovely and we soon settled in, we had to downsize a little which meant getting rid of quite a bit of stuff but that wasn't a problem as I took what we had got rid of to Hemswell car boot and luckily sold most of it.

The apartment was also a lot nearer to my lock up and it wasn't long before I was on the internet looking for a new project, and one evening as I trolled through eBay, Shpock and all the other sites, there on Gumtree was a quad bike for sale, and it was only in hull which is only about 30 minutes from where I live, so I messaged the guy and made arrangements to go and look it over that weekend. That Sunday I went to have a look at the quad which had been stood outside for quite a while and was rather tatty but for £130 you got what you paid for and I was soon squeezing it into the back of my estate car, luckily it just fit in. Upon getting home Linda thought I was barmy as it was in such a state but as I explained to her, that was the point of buying one to renovate. Over the next few weeks I stripped it down to the frame then started rubbing it down ready for painting then did the same with the plastic body panels and when they were all prepped and ready I sprayed the frame black and all the panels I did in a metallic blue, with three coats of clear and a good buff up I was very pleased with the finish I got. Next, I did the brakes and soon had the wheels back on which left me with the engine to sort out. I had decided not to put the same engine back in and put in a 125cc engine that I already had in the garage, with a few minor alterations I got it to fit.

Over the next few weeks I started getting a lot of pain in my left knee and soon found myself at Spires hospital in Anlaby Hull where I was told that it wasn't my knee that was the problem, it was my hip which was totally knackered and would need replacing ASAP. Arrangements were made for me to be admitted and given a new hip on the 9th of February 2019, well I had already had three knee replacements so the thought of a hip didn't bother my in the slightest as hip operations were not as complicated as knees and recovery time was a lot quicker, which is usually between 4-6 weeks, and this time I had the added bonus of the lovely Linda to bed bath me lol.

Then one day Linda asked me to find somewhere of my own to live, I was devastated but she had made her mind up and there was no changing it. She explained that it wasn't me, she just liked her own space but that didn't make me feel any better as I thought the marriage was over. As we talked, she said that we could still be married but just live in separate houses and still do things together that we did before, but it had hit me hard and I didn't know what to think anymore. Initially my mind was working overtime, had she got someone else, was she telling the truth, but Linda would always tell the truth even if offended, so I had to put them crazy ideas right out of my head. It wasn't easy as I blamed myself and no matter what I still loved her more then I could ever put into words, so I had to just go along with it and see what happens.

It wasn't long before I looked at a flat which was only around the corner from where Linda was, and it was the same Landlord which made moving much easier. The flat was nice so at the end of the month I moved in, and true to her word we still did the same things together as before but just slept in different places and if I'm been honest we got on a lot better, it wasn't ideal, well not for me as I didn't like living on my own, but Linda did and if it made her happy that's all that matters to me. It took a few weeks for me to get used to the new arrangements but as we were getting on so much better I soon got the gist of where she was coming from when she first mentioned it, but occasionally the little green monster in my head would pop up and drive me crazy but I soon learnt to pop him back in his box before I went totally round the bend. After a month in the flat, the one opposite became vacant so I went to have a look around and happy days it was nicer than mine and bigger, so I said I would have it, the landlord said he would have it decorated before I moved in and the guy moving out said he would shampoo all the carpets before he went, so that was me sorted for moving in hopefully at the beginning of April.

As soon as the decorating was done I started to move my stuff in and it wasn't long before I had it looking really nice, which was ok but as soon as it was done I was bored again.

I went down to the bedroom and put my mucky clothes on and went down to my garage where the quad bike was still waiting to be finished off, it only wanted the wiring sorted out, but it certainly had me baffled and after a good three hours I gave in and went home. The next day I was back at the garage having one more go, but the wiring on the quad was a bit of a bodge up with all the different coloured wires so it was really hard to follow anything or make any sense of the bloody Chinese wiring.

So after a further three hours I was still in the same position as yesterday (nowhere) when I decided enough was enough and called John in Wootton and asked him if he would do it for me, "certainly" he said "we can bring it over here and I'll soon have it sorted", oh happy days, I should have asked him in the first place, but if you don't try you'll never learn, ummm, well at least I'd tried and learnt sod all, but at least I had a go.

That weekend I had been to Huddersfield and had just gotten back into Goole when I spotted Linda walking by ASDA so I pulled over and asked her what she was up to, "not a lot, just looking in the shops" she replied, "well in that case do you fancy a coffee?" I asked, "Yes, that would be nice Nige", "ok then you save a table and I'll go get them".

For a good two hours we just sat and nattered about anything, it was pretty obvious to both of us that we still had feelings, for each other, and after all we were still married, she then said about trying again.

The next day I was receiving horrible texts, and in the last one she told me never to speak to her again or go anywhere near her, and she never said about trying again. Oh well, what the fuck, I was used to been treated like a twat by now, but it never gets any easier. I gave her want she wanted and left her alone and I never heard anything from her until I was sat writing this book a few weeks ago, when she messaged me asking if I fancied a coffee, "yes that would be nice" I replied "I'll be there in five minutes". After a coffee and a catch up we had decided to go out together in the morning, I was up bright and early, showered and getting ready for our outing when she texted me saying it was all over and never to speak to her again. Well where the fuck did that come from because I haven't got a clue what goes through her mind.

As you go through life just remember this book, because certain consequences can last a lifetime and I'm still living it every day.

After forty odd years of battling for each and every step that I've taken, there have been many times when I just wanted to close my eyes and never open them again, but that would have been a cop out, and far too easy, so I just carried on regardless of what I was told or what was suggested to me. The road I chose to go down has been a very long one with many stumbles along the way, not only did I prove the specialists wrong with what I have achieved, I surprised myself with just how far and how hard I was willing to push myself to get where I wanted to be.

When I look back to when I was lying in Lincoln intensive care with not a lot to live for, and then when I had been transferred to Huddersfield HRI where upon coming around I was given the low down on my condition, well if I say so myself, I think I've come a hell of a long way, from a paralysed crumpled mess lying in a hospital bed with not a lot to live for, to the qualified fitness instructor who also won two major star awards, one regional and one national, qualified to OCR standards as well as YMCA qualifications in teaching clients with disabilities and then shortlisted to carry the Olympic torch, well I think that's pretty impressive by any standards.

As for my personal life, well what can I say, all I ever wanted was someone for me, but that's harder to find then movement in my legs, and at the present living on my own, will I ever find what I'm looking for? Who knows?

So was the lifetime battle for fitness worth it? Oh god yes, did I have fun along the way? Oh god yes, and do I wish I had never got on a motorbike? Oh god no.

I wish things had been a lot different of course, but I have met a lot of very nice people along the way, and I can't praise the NHS enough for all they have done, and still doing for me.

It's amazing what you can achieve when you've got to, set your sights on your goals and go for it, don't let anyone or anything get in your way or talk you out of it.

There is a job to be done, so just get on with it.

Its now July 2019 and I'm now 62 years of age. My battle for fitness is still on going and over the last 3-4 weeks my leg has been a bastard when it comes to bedtime. As soon as my head hits the pillow either the left leg or the right starts to jump but strangely never both at the same time, and this is not just a twitch, oh no, it's a full blown muscle spasm and boy is it painful. Its so annoying as there is no chance of getting to sleep with either leg thrashing around the bed, and usually it goes on all night and bizarrely always stops around 6am the next day, by which time I am totally knackered, both physically and mentally.

The question I ask myself is why does it never affect both legs at the same time? And why does it only happen at night? And why does it stop around the same time the next morning? I've had every medication known to man, but nothing works, I've lost count of the specialists I have seen, but no one asks the same questions as me.

My last visit was to Hull royal where the specialist looked at me, then glanced at my notes then said there was nothing that could be done and I would just have to live with it (what the hell) how can they say this when they don't seem to know why it happens in the first place, and would she put up with it? I don't think so. If they could be bothered to admit me for a couple of nights, have me wired up for when the spasms start, they should be able to track the activity, find out where it comes from and then hopefully why it happens, but will they? Will they fuck and why? MONEY, if the government put as much money into the NHS as they waste on pointless tasks and oversea aid, perhaps our NHS wouldn't be struggling as much as it is (rant over).

I know with age we all deteriorate, but am I going to give in gracefully? ha not on your life, in the last six months I have been sent for more medicals by the government to justify why I am disabled, and this is after having mobility taken off me twice then reinstalled after a battle and taking it to court. Life can be hard, but don't be beaten, the road can be long but keep on walking and never doubt yourself out of what you want to achieve because there are plenty that will. And finally, if you have a goal in life, go for it, and never doubt your own ability because there is always some bastard somewhere that will.

In the end life can throw all kinds of shit your way, but you have to be quick and dodge it as sometimes you can get bogged down with it all, and if your not careful it will take you under. I thought I was a strong-willed person with all I have been through, but when Linda asked me to move out my confidence took a nosedive.

So right now, I'm sat here with a towel wrapped around my arm soaking up the blood from where I have cut myself as I have totally had enough.

I guess that would've been the easy way out, and luckily, I made a complete mess of it and just ended up with a very messed up arm (and head). Now

I feel like a total first-class twat, but in my defence your honour I was as low as you can get and it just seemed like the best way out, and since I've just had a really lovely day with Linda I'm so glad that I failed in what I was trying to achieve.

Where the hell do I go from here? Who knows because I certainly don't, I sometimes wish I could walk away but I can't no matter what, I totally love the woman even though the situation is slowly killing me. I don't know what to do, what to say, where to go, I think most days I don't even know what fucking day it is anymore. I'm sure I deserve better than a life where I am treated like something that she has stood in.

Anyway, back to the story. During my times in hospital I've had my share of operations, I've had so many on my femur to rebuild my right leg, then there was the operation to put a pin through my knee, there were three crucial ligament operations as well as quite a few operations to clean the knee out and draw fluid from it. Then later on I had three total knee replacements as well as a new hip and my leg shortening, as well as my nose rebroken and set, and now I'm told I could be having injections in my spine which should hopefully stop the leg spasms (hopefully) because this not sleeping thing is driving me around the twist.

BUT AT THE END OF THE DAY ALL I WANT IS MY WIFE BACK! NOT A LOT TO ASK FOR (WELL I DON'T THINK SO).

Over the last 42 years I have had to fight for every step I have taken and more so in the last 20 years as with age comes deterioration, but still the powers that be still insist on sending me for medicals in case over night I a miraculous recovery, but the thick bastards are totally brain dead when it comes to the facts, that when I could work, I did.

Gym instructor completes circuit on crutches and raises £200 for charity

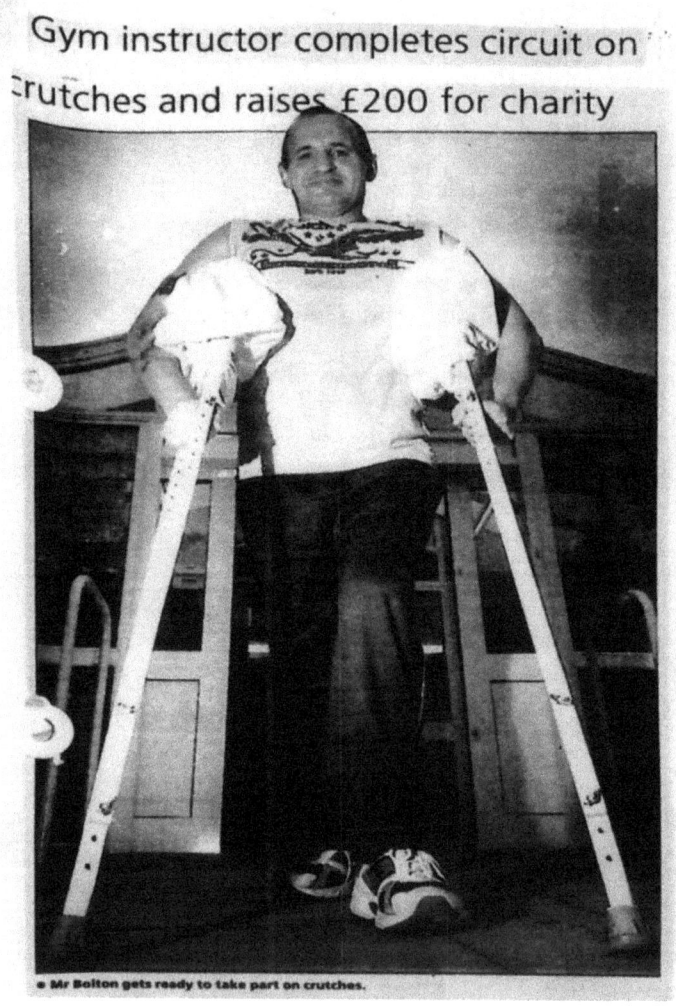

Gym instructor completes circuit on crutches and raises £200 for charity

● Mr Bolton gets ready to take part on crutches.

- Mr Bolton gets ready to take part on crutches.

**THE LION HEART
AWARD**

given to

NIGEL BOLTON

for being an inspiration to others.

**NOMINATED TO CARRY THE OLYMPIC FLAME IN
THE LONDON 2012 OLYMPIC TORCH RELAY BY**

Mr N Bolton

Not only did I work but I did a job that initially everyone thought was out of my capabilities due to my accident, WRONG, not only did I qualify to OCR levels I also got a YMCA qualifications in teaching fitness to clients with disabilities.

In my first year of college I won student of the year, then a little after that in 2009 I won two LSIS star awards which is the learning and skills improvement service where I gained one reginal and one national award for what I had achieved in my own life and what I had put back into my job as a fitness instructor.

Then in 2012 I was nominated to carry the Olympic torch for being an inspiration to others, not bad for a thick twat that only went to secondary modern school.

I must say that during my time in the Grimsby institute I had so much help and support from my co-workers which in the long term helped me gain the above, and I must also say that you would never find a better bunch of people. You know who you are, so I would like to take this opportunity to say thank you, thank you, thank you for giving me the opportunity to work with such talented, dedicated lovely people, it was a pleasure and I will never forget.

Thank you for making my life and world a far better place to be in.

Right now I'm sat writing this with kitchen towel roll wrapped around my arm soaking up the blood, what blood I hear you say, well it's the blood from where I have cut up my arm as I have totally had enough, so went for the easy way out, but as per usual I couldn't even get that right, hence why I'm sat here telling you about it and feeling rather down.

Now I have to find some way of hiding it until it heals up, yep I'm a first-class twat, but now I know why I couldn't cut that pork chop last week. I know it wasn't really fair as some poor bugger would have to find my body, and just think of the mess on the carpet, so now I have my mojo back and firing on all cylinders, things don't look that bad, but just for a short while my entire world came crashing down and I felt more cornered then I ever had before, and for the first time ever I couldn't cope.

Then I got to thinking, after all I had been through over the years and to come out of it walking and talking, then to end to end it like this? NOT ON YOUR FUCKING LIFE, and that's when I threw the knife into the sink, mopped up the blood and wrapped kitchen roll around my arm, and yes I'm a bloody idiot, but at least I have an excuse, a hemiparesis, a traumatic brain injury. In all the years since my accident, through all the operations and the battle to regain my mobility, never ever have I let it get me down, but I guess we all must have a cut-off point, and I think that day was mine. I suppose that after all the crap I had been through and four marriages its got to affect ones sanity in some way, but what the fuck, I'm still here and here to stay (it was just a wobble) and I intend to enjoy the rest of my life to the full as it took a hell of a lot to get where I am without cutting it short with some mindless act of self-butchery. So I hope you enjoyed your read and perhaps learnt a few things along the way, and hopefully by now you may have a different outlook on life.

After all that had happened over the last few months, like moving out and getting my own place because Linda wanted it, getting on with my own life because Linda wanted it and meeting someone else because Linda wanted it. For quite a while I was adamant that I didn't want anyone else, I only wanted my wife back, but she wasn't having any of it and told me to find someone as she wasn't coming back and it would make things a lot easier on myself. In the end there's only so long you can put your life on hold until you realise that things aren't going to change so I did exactly what she told me to do and met someone else, but what the fuck, I was still wrong, apparently I did it too quick, but I got on with my life and it was doing ok until the day I bumped into Linda on my way home, we talked without arguing which was a bonus and then made the biggest mistake ever, instead of going with my heart, my head took over and we both agreed to try again, and that's when she said "you must finish with her first".

The next day I made the phone call that ended it, but when I mentioned it to Linda she said she had never asked me to do it or agreed to trying again, so now I was left with fuck all and deep down I think she did it purposely, over the next few weeks life just carried on as usual until one day we went out together, and ended up in the pub. After drinking quite a few gins we made our way back to her flat where we had coffee and talked.

I said I didn't like it on my own and she said I didn't need to be on my own, I could spend all day tomorrow with her if I wanted, "oh thanks" I replied "but I guess I better make my way home" "ok then I'll see you tomorrow" she said as I walked out the door, "just text me when you get home", "ok I will" I replied as I made my way to the lift.

The next morning I was up and on quite early getting ready to go to Linda's for the day when I received a text, it was from Linda, she said it's over so leave me alone and I am not going to change my mind and I don't want any kind of relationship with you, and don't try to change my mind. Well you know when you're about to explode? Umm I was about there, I was sick of been treated like something she had stood in and only talking to me when she could be bothered. I ain't a bad guy and I deserve a lot better than to be treated this way, I had taken as much shit as I was going to take, I don't know what goes through her brain, but if it were up to me she would be committed.

After all that had gone on between us, I still loved her because when she wasn't been a twat, she was a lovely person and lovely to be with. So as Sunday loomed up, I asked her if she fancied doing something. "Yes" she replied "that would be nice" so on Sunday morning I picked her up and we went for a walk around Selby.

After a couple of hours, I asked if she wanted any lunch "yep, ok, then where are we going to go?" "if we drive back to yours and park the car we can walk to Wetherspoons" I replied, "good idea Nige, see your not that thick" she said as she got into the car.

Thirty minutes later we were sat at a table eating lunch and knocking back the gins with a splash of lemonade, and after lunch there were more gins, then more gins and even more gins and by now we were both pretty liquored up so decided to walk back to her apartment and have coffee. As we sat, we talked about our predicament I said that I didn't like been on my own, to which Linda replied "you can spend the day here tomorrow with me, if you want?" "yes, that would be lovely thanks, but I guess I should make my way home" and as I walked through the door, she said "see you tomorrow".

The next day I was up and showered and ready for off when I got a text, it was from Linda, and it said, we are over, I don't want a relationship with you or anything else, just leave me alone, don't call or bother me again. Well where the fuck had that come from? She had pushed me as far as I was going to be pushed, so I let her get on with it and didn't go anywhere near her. Then one day as I was sitting in the library writing this book, she texted me and asked if I wanted a coffee, "yes that would be nice" I replied, "I'll be there in a few minutes".

When I got there, she gave me a coffee and a few dirty looks but was I bothered? Not on your life, "so I thought you didn't want anything more to do with me" I asked, "well I missed you and this mess is my fault as I don't try hard enough", "ok then, but where do we go from here?" I replied. "well we try harder Nige, if that's what you want that is?" I know she was a twat, but she was my twat and I knew what she was like.

It is now Tuesday 22nd of August, Linda has gone for her hair doing and I'm sat finishing this book, on Monday we went to Bournemouth for four days and sharing the same room which will be a big test for Linda, but me and my friend the gin bottle will be there to keep her company.

Do I think it's going to work? I don't know. I will give it 100%, you can bet your life on that one.

CONCLUSION

Even though I've tried to cover most things but due to my head injury there are things that I have forgotten which sometimes come back to me, like the time I went to Spain after on holiday shortly after getting married the first time. On arrival at the Spanish airport we discovered that the country was in the middle of a heat wave which at the time pleased me as we were guaranteed good weather. But by the end of the first week I was in agony with my knee, due to the heat the metal pieces I had were expanding and the pain was unbelievable, so a lot of the time I could be found sat on the pool side dangling my leg in the water to keep the damn thing cool. Unfortunately upon returning home I discovered that with it expanding and then cooling down it had not gone back to where it started out, so consequently everything else was out of line and it wasn't long before I was going back in to get it sorted out.

After that operation it was like starting again and it took quite a few months to get back to where I had been, but hey it wasn't anything new, five steps forward and three steps back.

Then we fast forward to the present day and the ongoing battle with the government policies and all the red tape, and yet again I have to go for further medical to justify my condition, I have for the first time found out what it is called which is hemiparesis which is a traumatic brain injury, and after I had googled the word I frightened myself to death at what I was reading.

The side effects of the condition are enough to have you committed to a nut house, and I always knew that after my second accident I had changed (somehow) but after reading the list below, this was definitely me:

- Spasticity
- Contractures
- Shoulder pain
- Foot drop
- Muscle weakness to one side of the body
- Irritable
- Short temper
- Speech difficulties
- Behavioural problems
- Muscle seizures

But what the hell, like I've said before you just get on with it, because it you don't, nobody is going to do it for you. They say that its nonprogressive, ha fucking idiots, with age you start deteriorating and you get worse, so if that isn't a type of progression, I don't know what the hell is.

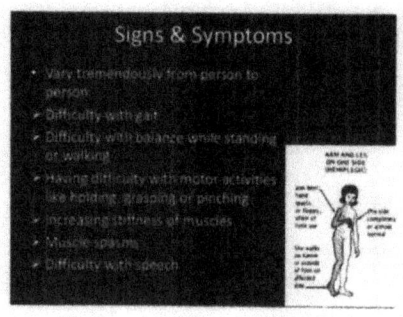

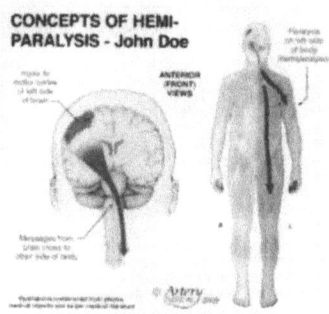

After breaking up with Brenda, Linda said she never mentioned that we would try again, and over the next few months no matter what I suggested she didn't want to do it or didn't want to go anywhere with me. At the same time she talked to me and treated me like shit, but I guess I was at fault for putting up with it and at the same time she let her overweight goby friend slag me off, who actually knows bugger all about me, but she never put her straight or told her the truth.

I suggested lots of things, even going to Italy as I knew it was somewhere that she wanted to go but all I got was "whatever" there's only so low you can go! And I was rock bottom. I just wanted to die and put an end to all the torment I was going through, she had to do what two motorbike accidents and all that I had been through over the years had failed to do, she had broken me and I was a mess. The only person who got what they wanted was her, it was all me me me, and then a few weeks ago I was busily looking for a holiday to Italy when she said "IT'S OVER, I don't want anything else to do with you, not even friends, and it would be better if you didn't talk to me either", well where the fuck did that come from? Who knows what goes on in her brain? So that's just what I did, because by now I had totally lost the plot and had enough so just let her get on with it. But I got to thinking, what hell is it me? Am I such a bad bastard that no one wants me?

Eventually I picked myself up and went on a few dates, but my heart wasn't in it at all. I went on one date and all she talked about for three hours was herself, and how pretty she was, until I couldn't stand it anymore and got up, made my excuses and left, but even then she shouted after me "don't you want to see me again", "no" I replied "your bloody boring" then I got into my car and left.

After a bit of time on my own my life settled down, I still keep going on dates but not found the right one yet, I've got one this weekend (fingers crossed) but I'd rather be on my own then make another mistake, and that's about the lot. I hope you have enjoyed reading about my life, I bet reading about it was easy, living through it was a bloody nightmare, but hey I'll get there one day.

And finally, will there be a follow on to this book?

You bet there will.

Lightning Source UK Ltd.
Milton Keynes UK
UKHW010624270722
406441UK00001B/44